Medicinal 1

Includes Aromatherapy, Essential Oils, And Herbal Medicines To Improve Your Health

J.J Ortezky

Table of Contents

INTRODUCTION 7
HISTORY OF THE HERBS 12
CHEMISTRY OF THE HERBS 20
    Alkaloids 20
    Tannins 21
    Cardiac glycosides 22
    Saponins 24
    Anthraquinones 26
    Flavonoids 26
    Essential oils 27
    Vegetable oils 29
    Bitter principles 29
    Mucilages 30
    Organic acids 30
    Vitamins and trace elements 31
ALTERNATE METHODS OF ALTERNATE MEDICINE 32
    ACUPUNCTURE 32
    THE ALEXANDER TECHNIQUE 35
    AUTOGENIC TRAINING 37
    AYURDVEDIC MEDICINE 38
    CHIROPRACTICE 39
    CHINESE MEDICINE 40
    COLOUR THERAPY 42
    HYDROTHRAPY 43

- KINESIOLOGY 44
- MASSAGE 45
- REFLEXOLOGY 46
- REIKI 47
- SHIATSU 48
- AROMATHERAPY 50
- HOMEOPATHY 51

PREPARATION OF THE POTIONS 54
- Infusions 57
- Decoctions 57
- Tinctures 57
- Glycerol 58
- Fluid extracts 58
- Syrups 59
- Powders 59
- Pills 59
- Baths 60
- Ointments 60
- Poultices 61
- Compresses 61
- Plasters 62

DISPOSABLE INDISPOSITIONS AND THEIR HERBAL TREATMENTS 63
- Common cold 64
- Catarrh 66
- Sore throat 67
- Coughs 68

Indigestion	70
Diarrhea	71
High blood sugar	73
High cholesterol and heart health	74
Urinary tract infections	74
Joint pain and arthritis	75
Cancer prevention	75
PRINCIPLES OF HERBAL MEDICINE	76
HERB ACTIONS	88
HEALING HERBS	93

INTRODUCTION

Herbalists and herbalism have often been underestimated. In fact, herbalism is thought to be a mere collection of home-made granny recipes, which are to be used occasionally and sparingly for harmless ailments like the common cold. For many, resorting to herbs for treatment of diseases is an obsolete tradition and has no place in today's world of magic medicines. Little do they know that every medicinal drug today, under all that sophisticated vacuum packing and austere form, is a refined derivative of some sort of herbal plant.

This century however, has been much kinder to herbalists. Especially the past couple of decades; herbal medicine has emerged as a very effective alternate to conventional allopathic medicine. Today, you will find that the most sophisticated of medical stores will also have a section dedicated solely to over-the-counter herbal preparations. Apart from pharmacists, beauticians have also turned to 'natural' beauty products; you will find that currently the hottest selling shampoos, soaps and cosmetics are those which identify their nature as being purely organic. One of the best examples of the growing popularity of herbs can be seen in the success of The Body Shop® and its pure natural products. Even gourmet chefs refuse to be left behind in the pursuit of naturality; you will find that recently the best culinary spices and garnishes are fresh herbs.

The World Health Organization had made an announcement in the 70's where they claimed that the only way we can achieve an appropriate standard of health care in the world by the millennium is, if Third World countries resort to their traditional systems of medicine rather than wait for the modern world of healthcare to come rescue them. In fact, many first world countries have turned to herbal medicine and have started recognizing its benefits.

The French have led the way in the eighties by inaugurating the first chair of herbal medicine in the University of Paris North; Britain and the United states have started conducting research trials on the effects of herbal medicine and Germany is now the largest manufacturer of phyto-pharamceuticals. German homeopathic medicines are exported to countries throughout the world.

The properties of certain herbs like ginseng, garlic, evening primrose oil and devil's claw have been recognized and published in many research papers. Currently, there is great international interest in exploring plants which boost the immune system.

No doubt, the eventual abandonment of synthetic chemical foods and medicines is a consequence of the 'green' revolution; still it is the unmistakable healing power of these natural elements that are drawing people towards themselves.

Unfortunately, there is still insufficient organization related to academics and practice in this field. The only reason why herbalists from Europe can combat with modern western medical doctors is because of the perseverance and dedication of a few individuals who inherited knowledge related to this field from their parents who inherited from their ancestors. Examples of certain such personalities include the famous Maurice Mességué, who learnt from his father. Similarly, Britain's leading herbalist, F. Fletcher Hyde, who was also the President Emeritus of the National Institute of Medical Herbalists, was student and predecessor to his father and was himself succeeded by both his sons.

The United States of America, on the other hand, gave a tough time to this realm of medicine. Rather it was the American Medical Association which took the initiative initially to wipe out this 'obsolete' field of study. It was only due to certain religious groups like the Mormons and the Seven-Day Adventurists that herbal medicine managed to stick around in this region.

Today however, there is an army of dedicated herbalists who have helped establish full time schools of herbal medicine and clinics. The other branches of alternate medicine are also given their due worth of respect and students are offered several areas of expertise to train in, including Chinese Herbal medicine, Ayurvedic medicine and Tibetan herbal traditions, among many others that have been mentioned later in this book.

Although many plants are in common, they are often used for different purposes. For example, herbalists in China use the hawthorn berries for helping with digestion, whereas, Western herbalists used them as a tonic for heart conditions and regulating blood pressure. Although slightly different, there is an overlap between the practice of herbal medicine in different regions; but one is certain: the repetitive success and results of various plant extracts throughout the world have proved to be as convincing as research trials that these miracle plants are truly a precious gift from nature.

The way forward now is to use herbal medicine in its entirety as well as complementary to modern medicine. The two may be different but they are most definitely not mutually exclusive. You can't possibly separate the two; it would be like separating the mother from her children. Herbal medicine is undoubtedly the mother of modern medicine.

And the end of all our exploring
Will be to arrive where we started
And know the place for the first time
- *T.S. Eliot, Little Gidding*

HISTORY OF THE HERBS

The art of using herbs for medicinal purposes is perhaps as old as mankind itself. During the earliest civilizations, people used to consume certain plants with their food so as to derive benefit from them. It has been found by remains of tablets that during the ancient Sumerian period, dating back as far as 3500 BC, wounds were dressed with a particular 'ointment' which was made by heating animal fat or plant resin with some sort of alkali. This mixture yielded a soapy consistency and had antibiotic properties. There is very frequent mention of use of sesame oil, also for antibacterial purposes.

The next prominent civilization after the Sumerians is the Egyptian civilization. Slave workers in ancient Egypt are said to have been given a certain ration of garlic, onions and radishes to eat daily so as to help prevent fevers and infections. In fact, the very first written records of herbs and their benefits have been found to belong to the ancient Egyptians. Most of the knowledge today, about the use of herbs, can be traced back to Egyptian priests who used to practice herbal medicine. Records have been found dating back to 3000 BC, wherein herbs such as caraway and cinnamon have been mentioned. To date, the Egyptians of that era are considered as most knowledgeable and skillful when it comes to the use of herbs. This is further reinforced by the fact that a comprehensive record of the Eber's Papyrus, written back in 1500 BC, is intact till today; herein are mentioned the names of some 700 herbal remedies which the Egyptians were familiar with and used regularly.

The Eber's Papyrus is has been recorded in such that great detail that even particulars such as how to administer treatments and in what form have been mentioned. These herbs included thyme, onion, parsley and balsam apple for *pain relief*; honey milk and sesame for *asthma;* mint, garlic, juniper and sandalwood as *digestive aids;* mint and caraway as *breath freshener;* mustard seeds, aloe and juniper for *chest pains;* aloe for burns n skin diseases. Some of the 'recipes' for these remedies, as ridiculous as they sound, have been mentioned below:

<u>Hairwash for the Queen Shesh of Egypt</u>

- *The claw of a dog- 1/3 part*
- *Decayed palm leaves-1/3 part*
- *The hoof- 1/3 part*

Boil in oil and massage into head.

For Treatment of diarrhea

- *Spring onions*
- *Groats recently boiled*
- *Oil and honey*
- *Wax and water*

Boil together, drink for four days.

Moving further on, during the time of the Indus Valley Civilisation, between 3000 BC and 300 BC, the Indians made their contributions to the field of medicines by writing books on herbal medicine by the names of *Charak Samhita* and *Susrut Samhita* and translating them into other languages such as Arabic. Thereby influencing the Persians, Arabs and to some extent even Greeks with their infinite knowledge of natural healing. Perhaps the people of the time gained their knowledge from the Hindu scriptures revealed at the time. For example, there is mention of 'Soma' a Vedic ritual drink in the *Rigveda*, a prominent Hindu scripture. Not just here, but this plant is also mentioned in the *Avesta*, the sacred text of the Zoroastrians. After much speculation about the identity of the 'Soma' plant, it has been found to belong to the family *Ephedra*. It would be fair to say that the herbalists of the Indus Civilisation have laid the foundations for today's Ayurvedic medicine

The doctors of Babylon, in 1900 BC, inherited most of their knowledge from Sumerians. However, they made some contributions to this field on their own as well.

The *materia medica* of the Babylonian physicians includes mention of saltpeter as an astringent and salt as an antiseptic. Other natural substances they used abundantly include milk; thyme; willow; pear; fir; figs; dates; snakeskin; turtle-shell; cassia and myrtle. They usually prepared their medicines by boiling them in water with alkali & salts and administering them as concoctions.

The great Assyrian herbal, coined from some 40,000 different stone tablets is proof enough of how rampant the practice of herbal medicine was in this era. These tablets date back to 1100 BC, a time when the Greek civilization was also at its peak. These fragments of knowledge engraved in stone were found during excavation of ruins of the Temples at Nineveh. After a painstaking compilation, it has been found that this collection amounts to names of about a thousand plants which were used during the Sumerian and Assyrian periods. This proves, that many herbal names today are derivatives of their counterparts from the ancient Sumerian language. Some of these names have undergone minor changes, taking influence from the Greeks and Arabs, who also were generous in their use of these herbs. When we pronounce names like saffron, cardamom, turmeric, cumin, carob, mulberry , myrrh, flax, cherry, almond, sesame, poppy, mandrake, lupin and cypress, we are not speaking English, rather a dialect of the language of ancient Sumerians!

The Greeks, much like their counterparts, the Arabs, mostly inherited their medical knowledge from the Egyptians. In fact, they identified Egyptian gods as the very first physicians and herbalists; they regarded Asclepius, the Egyptian god of medicine, to be the son of Apollo, the sun god. Many schools of medicine were established during the Greek period, the founders of these schools, including the renowned Greeks Pythagoras and Hippocrates, were tutored by Egyptian priests. This knowledge was further transferred down to Ancient Rome, in 700 BC.

Dioscorides, official doctor to the Roman armies during the reign of emperors Clauduis and Nero, travelled a wide expanse of the world while on duty, and was able to gather an immense amount of knowledge regarding herbs. Dioscorides then compiled all his first-hand knowledge in the form of a book, *De Materia Medica.* This is the ultimate compilation of herbal medicine which was the benchmark for many professional herbalists to come. The authenticity of this book can be gauged from the fact that this was the standard medical textbook for civilized nations for more than thirteen centuries after it was compiled. Even doctors of the Turkish Empire, in the 19th century had great regard for this book and its matter.

To say that the Romans were influenced by the Holy Bible, would be an understatement. It is during the Roman period that the Bible was revealed and compiled. There are many herbs mentioned in different verses of the Holy Bible, in the Song of Solomon and Exodus.

There are many passages where the healing qualities of many herbs have been mentioned. Some fourteen herbs that have been mentioned in the Bible are listed below:

- Aloe Vera
- Anise
- Balm
- Bitter Herbs (include lettuce, horseradish, coriander seeds, horehound, endive and tansy)
- Cassia
- Cinnamon
- Cumin
- Frankincense
- Garlic
- Hyssop
- Mint
- Mustard
- Myrrh
- Saffron

The physician to the Roman Emperor and Philosopher Marcus Aurelius, famous for being a healer himself, was Claudius Galen. Claudius was the author of the herbal *De Simplicibus,* the final compilation of all herbal knowledge inherited from the Greeks and beyond.

This compilation by Claudius was used religiously by the Arabs, among other Greek herbals, and formed the foundation of the medical school at Cairo which was established *much* later in the thirteenth century by Abdullah Ibn Al-Baitar, a famous Arab botanist.

The Arab civilization was in the shadows until 700 AD, after the Holy Quran was revealed and Islam started spreading far and wide into the world. The Arab medical specialists combined previous knowledge handed down by the Egyptians and the previous scriptures with the herbs mentioned in the Quran. One such verse is in chapter 13 of the Holy Quran:

'..and in the earth there are tracts side by side and gardens of corn and grapes and palm trees having one root and (others) having distinct roots-- they are watered with one water, and we make some of them excel others in fruit; most surely there are signs in this for a people who understand..'

Certain herbs of immense healing properties mentioned in the Quran are:

- Olives and olive oil
- Garlic
- Onions
- Ginger
- Dates
- Figs
- Milk
- Honey

And so did Herbal medicine see consequent eras of Henry VIII in the early 16th century; Sir Walter Raleigh and his herbals published in1597; Paracelsus of the late 16th century and his theory ' *it only depends upon the dose whether the poison is a poison or not',* successfully discovering the remedies of *Cinchona succirubra* for malaria, *Cephaelis Ipecacuanha* for dysentery and *Smilax Ornata* for syphilis; Reverend Edward Stone and his concoctions of aspirin and salicylic acid for Rheumatism in 1763; 'New Domestic Herbal' of John Waller in 1822 to the origin of The National Association of Medical Herbalists in Britain, 1864, which is functional to date under the name of National Institute of Medical Herbalists.

CHEMISTRY OF THE HERBS

Modern science has done more than its part in identifying and isolating chemicals from plants and processing and packaging them to serve as the 'miracle pills' that today's medicine is so dependent upon. There have been researches upon researches that have been conducted and almost all the relevant ones published. All this information can only benefit herbalists and help them understand their plants better. However, despite all science and research, time and again it has been proved that these working chemicals alone do not achieve the desired results as does using the *whole* plant. The chemicals that have been identified serve the sole purpose of helping us understand how the herbs work. Some of the active chemicals are mentioned below:

Alkaloids

As a rule of thumb, all alkaloids contain nitrogen. The derived their names when some scientists discovered them and thought them to be plant alkalis. The world today, is more than familiar with some prominent alkaloids: nicotine, caffeine and morphine to name a few. The characteristic quality of alkaloids is that they have a profound effect on the central nervous system. Like many drugs, alkaloids taste very bitter. One of the first alkaloids discovered was Narcotine; it was isolated from the opium poppy back in the early nineteenth century. An interesting fact is that alkaloid levels in plants vary in accordance with the time of the day, month and even year! They are said to attain the highest concentration just before they are about to flower. Alkaloids have been found to be a major constituent in many medicinal plants. However, the effect of a combination of different alkaloids, as they are present in plants is very difficult to determine. The results obtained are strikingly different to those obtained by simply administering isolated alkaloids.

Tannins

Tannins are used, surprisingly, precisely as their name suggests. They are used to *tan* leather. This process is performed by using the bark of the oak tree, which is said to have very high tannin content. Tannin reacts with the protein present in animal skin and coagulates the protein such that is becomes resistant to putrefaction. Throughout the past centuries, tannin has been very useful to people. For example, tannin was used to make ink; the classical blue colour was attained by added iron salts to tannin solutions. Another benefit of tannin, which renders it extremely useful to wine makers till today is its ability to clear wine hazes. The tannins cause the proteins and other related substances in the wine to precipitate, hence rendering the wine 'clean'.

Tannins are abundant in nature, and are plentiful in plenty of plants. They are usually present in a very high concentration in the external most parts of the plant, like the bark for example. An interesting fact is that this location of tannin also has a purpose; to drive away predators.

Coming to our area of interest, the application of tannin in medicine started because of its astringent properties. Therefore many astringent herbs used on inflamed mucosa and wounds have high tannin content. The tannin causes an impermeable layer to form over the wound and hence help speed up healing. Therefore herbs containing tannin are used on cuts, minor burns, swellings, inflammation, hemorrhoids and even varicose veins. Herbalists have also found tannin to be very valuable on ingestion; it is an effective antidote for diarrhea, peptic ulcer and colon inflammation. However the preparation of tannin containing medicine is tricky as it undergoes a chemical reaction as soon as it comes in contact with air and becomes inert. Therefore plants containing tannins should not be stored for too long and should be used immediately.

Cardiac glycosides

Cardiac glycosides are nature's miracle drug for the heart. They have a structure consisting of a sugar group and a non-sugar group. It is the non-sugar group that is actually the active functional part of this chemical. However, as useless as the sugar group sounds, it is the compound responsible for the taking up of these glycosides by the heart. This supports our earlier claim of active components achieving complete efficacy only in the wholeness of their parent plant. Cardiac glycosides are abundant in many plants, especially those flourishing in European countries. These plants include foxglove (*Digitalis*), squills (*Urginea maritima*), lily of the valley (*Convallaria majalis*), wallflowers (*Cheiranthus cheiri*) and pheasants cyc (*Adonis vernulis*). This compound is also found in certain plants native to East and West Africa; this was well utilized by African tribesmen and they extracted the glycosides from the seeds of these plants to make arrow poison.

Today, the foxglove plant, also known as Digitalis, is an unmatchable phenomenon in the medical world. It yields the only drug, Digoxin, which supports weak hearts and is used in every other prescription for patients with failing hearts.

The cardiac glycosides are able to support a weak heart because they increase the strength of contraction of the cardiac muscle without requiring an increases supply of oxygen.

In contrast to allopathic medicine, herbal medicine prefers lily of the valley as a source for these glycosides as they are released slowly that those in the foxglove and are also efficiently excreted from the body, preventing any possible toxicity.

Saponins

Saponins can be said to belong to the family of glycosides. As the name suggests, they have the ability to achieve a soapy consistency once they come in contact with water. The first soap was manufactured by saponins extracted from the plant Soapwort (*Saponaria officinalis*). The incredible quality of the lather that is built up due to the soapy quality is very effective in removing dirt and grease off the skin.

Having said that, saponins are not always beneficial, in fact, if they enter the body via the wrong route, they can actually wreck havoc with the body. For instance, if saponins are injected directly into the blood they cause hemolysis i.e. breakdown of the red blood cells. However they are completely harmless when taken orally as they aren't absorbed at all. However they do aid the absorption of calcium and silicon from the intestines. Some common plants containing saponins are spinach, tomatoes, asparagus and oats.

Another quality that saponins are endowed with is that of being an expectorant. Expectoration occurs when saponins irritate nerve endings of the digestive tract and causes reflex coughing. Plants containing saponins which are commonly used expectorants are cowslip roots (*Primula veris*), mullein (*Verbascum thapsus*) , liquorice (*Glycyrrhiza glabra)* and sweet violet (*Violata odorata).*

The most captivating aspect of saponins is their similarity in structure, and hence functions, to the human hormones of sex and stress. These hormones are secreted by the adrenal gland and the reproductive organs i.e. the ovaries and testes. Other substances that saponins bear resemblance to are cholesterol, Vitamin D, estrogen and progesterone.

The plants which are rich in saponins mostly belong to the lily family including like sarsaparilla and trillium, and the Solonaceae family of plants, of which the woody-night shade (*Solanum dulcamara*) is often used.

Slightly different, but definitely related are triterpenoids. These are also saponins, although they have a different function and mode of action. Famous plants, like the oriental ginseng (*Panax ginseng*), owes its fame to these organic substances. Ginseng is known world over for its ability to normalize human hormone balance and also alleviate stress. This particular action on ginseng is referred to as adaptogenic effect.

Other herbs with hormone regulating saponins include black cohosh (*Cimicifuga racemosa*), blue cohosh (*Caulophyllum thalictroides*), false unicorn root (*Chamaelerium luteum*) and other sarsaparilla species. Saponins are extracted from plants like horse chestnut (*Aesculus hippocastanum*), liquorice and wild yam (*Dioscorea villosa*), for their anti-inflammatory action.

Anthraquinones

Anthraquinones are actually plant dyes, but are well known for their medicinal effects similar to glycosides. They have been used in the production of commercial dyes for ages and are mostly found in dyer's madder (*Rubia tinctorum).* The glycosidal action unique to anthraquinones is that they are effective laxatives. This laxative effect occurs when glycosides irritate the wall of the large bowel and increases its motility. Many herbs including senna, rhubarb, cascara, aloes, buckthorn and alder are well known and frequently used for their bowel evacuating properties. However, overuse can make the bowel too dependant on these substances and normal bowel habits will be altered.

Flavonoids

Flavonoids are also a sort of glycosides and appear in plants as well as in free state. The plant families Polygonacea, Leguminosae, Rutaceae, Compositae and Umbelliferae are said to abundant in flavonoids. These are also used as dyes as they have a very strong natural colour. The bright yellow colour of the cowslip is an example of the intensity of yellow given off by this substance. Flavonoids present in buchu (*Agathosma betulina)* and broom (*Sarothamnus scoparius*) are used a potent diuretics, whereas those present in liquorice (Glycyrrhiza glabra) and parsley areused as antispasmodics. Recently, flavonoids called rutin and hesperidin (formerly known as Vitamin P) have been said to act in synergy with Vitamin C and also increase the ability of the body to utilize vitamin C.

Most common uses of flavonoids are in treatment of bruising, post-partum bleedins and nose-bleeding as they strengthen the walls of blood vessels. Other properties associated with these organic chemicals are antibacterial, antiviral and antihypertensive.

Essential oils

Essential oils are essentially substances that are volatile, i.e. easily evaporated. Therefore their extraction hardly required any effort. They can be withdrawn from leaves by simply crushing them or even warming slightly under sunlight. These oils have a distinct fragrance which can be detected immediately due to their volatility. Some of more familiar essential oils include peppermint, where the actual oil is *menthol*; thyme, with the main oil as *thymol*; and sage having its main essential oil as *thujone.* The aroma that arises from certain plants is actually due to subtle combination of these essential oils; their different concentrations determining characteristic smells.

What's fascinating is that these oils, when oxidized, as happens in conifer trees, give rise to plant resins and gums.

Due to their unique nature, essential oils can easily get absorbed anywhere in the body. In fact, when inhaled through the nose, these oils can have an immediate effect on the brain. For instance, the scents of mint and rosemary are known to improve concentration and increase awareness. Essential oils are also known to help digestion, when taken orally. This is because they irritate the oral mucous membranes slightly, just enough to increase salivation.

Another distinctive quality of essential oils is that they stimulate the cardiovascular system, causing the heart to beat faster, the respiratory rate to rise and the circulation to become more efficient. Essential oils have also been known for their use as diaphoretics, because they are excreted from the skin; as diuretics because they are also excreted by the kidneys and expectorants because partial excretion is via the lung as well.

Another advantage of these substances is that they have antiobiotic and germicidal properties, especially, allicin from garlic and thymol from thyme.

While preparing to take essential oils, the plants containing them must not be boiled because they will evaporate in no time. Also once prepared, all precautions must be taken to lock in the steam otherwise the actual aromatized content will be lost with the steam.

Once inhaled with steam, these oils help liquidate mucosal secretions and are extremely effective for congested sinuses, nose and chest. On external application, some oils such as clove oil, have an anesthetic effect. This is why clove oil is a well-known household remedy for toothache. Some oils, such as mustard oil are used for external application in rheumatic arthritis.

Vegetable oils

Vegetable are also oils, very similar to essential oils, with the only distinguishing factor being that they are *fixed* rather than *volatile.* Vegetable oils are unsaturated and preferred over animal fats which are saturated and more likely to block blood vessels leading to a stroke or heart attack. Some commonly tapped sources of vegetable oils include sunflower, coconut, canola, olive, cottonseed, palm, peanut, safflower, sesame and soybean.

Bitter principles

Bitters have very similar modes of action, albeit very diverse structures. The bitterness in these substances stimulates release of digestive juices in the stomach and also increases motility. Therefore, apart from aiding digestion, they help stimulate the appetite. Hence the reason why many people drink bitter apperitifs before having meals. Gentian root (*Gentiana lutia),* centaury (*centaurium erythraea)* and wormwood *(Artemisia absinthium),* are a few plants rich in bitters. Bitters make up a substantial portion of beer drinks.

Mucilages

Mucilages are also referred to as polysaccharides, which are long chains or sugars, which are grossly visible as slimy exudates of some plants. These strings of mucous actually swell when placed in water and make for an effective soothing gel. Mucilages are very good in retaining heat, hence their use as external hot compresses on abscesses and boils.

These are also very efficient in soothing damaged mucous membranes; therefore they are frequently used to heal ulcers. Some plants containing mucilages include marhsmallows (*Althaea officinalis*), comfrey (*Symphytum officinale*), linseed (*Linum usitatissimum*), psyllium seed (*Plantago psyllium*) and Irish moss (*Chondrus crispus*). Psyllium seeds and linseeds are commonly used as laxatives because they swell in water and make for a good amount of bulk.

Organic acids

Organic acids make up for an essential part of metabolism in the body. Examples include citric acids, malic acids and tartaric acids. These acids are present in high quantities in unripe fruits rather than ripe fruits. They are somewhat responsible for keeping these fruits fresh for a long time. Ascorbic acid, better known as Vitamin C, is widely present in a number of fruits, herbs and vegetables. Functions include antibacterial, laxative and diuretic properties.

However, all acids cannot be said to be good for health. Certain acids like oxalic acids, present in tomatoes, rhubarb and sorrel, can predispose certain people to kidney stones or an acute attack of gout.

Vitamins and trace elements

Nature has provided sources for a complete range of vitamins. Although vitamin D is an exception because this is mostly present in dairy products or manufactured within the skin on exposure to sunlight. Beta-carotene, also called provitamin A is a yellow pigment containing substance, which is converted to vitamin A by the liver. Nature is an abundant source for another very common vitamin which is vitamin C. There are innumerable fruits and vegetables full of these vitamins. Some of these herbs are dandelion, watercress, nettles and rosehips. Rosehips also have a substantial amount of iron content, which improves absorption of vitamin C. Trace elements include minerals like sodium and potassium, Dandelions are known as potent diuretics for their high potassium content.

ALTERNATE METHODS OF ALTERNATE MEDICINE

ACUPUNCTURE

Acupuncture is an art of Ancient China and involves the insertion of fine needles into skin at different locations of the body. It has said to date back to almost 2,500 years. The concept behind acupuncture is that there are flow patterns of energy, referred to as Qi, which are responsible for maintenance of a healthy body. The origin of any disease is due to a disruption in this flow of energy. Acupuncture is therefore used to restore this flow of energy at various points on the body.

Interestingly enough, the actual term 'Acupuncture' was first used by a Dutch physician, William Ten Rhyne, when he was living in Japan during the 17th century. He then introduced acupuncture to people in Europe. Acupuncture literally means 'to prick with a needle'.

The very first book on Acupuncture, *Nei Chin Su Wen (Yellow Empero's classic of Internal Medicine),* was written way back in 400 BC. It went on to become a very widely practiced approach in the 1800s; British soldiers preferred Acupuncture over all other forms of medicine for relief from fever and pain.

The points of the body along which these needles are inserted in are located alongside meridians. According to the Chinese tradition, the human body is composed of two forces: yin and yang. These two forces are quite well known as the black and white fish swimming in opposite directions. The yin and yang are said to be complementary yet opposite forces. The yin is the feminine force; calm and passive, and representing the cool moisture or darkness. The yang is the corresponding masculine force; aggressive and stimulating, representative of heat and light. Any illness is said to be due to an imbalance in these forces. For instance, a person with high blood pressure of severe headache is said to have an excess of yang, whereas a person with a feeling of tiredness, cold and fluid retention is representative of the female counterpart in this story.

It is needless to say that Acupuncture has more effect on certain types of diseases than it does on others. Therefore, the ailments which have more than just benefited from Acupuncture are mentioned below:

Diseases of the Muscles, Bones and Joints

- Rhematoid Arthritis
- Sprains
- Headaches
- Osteoarthritis

Diseases of the Nervous System

- Anxiety, Depression and Other Nervous Disorders
- Nerve Paralysis
- Other Nervous Diseases
- Strokes
- The Neuralgias

Disorders of the Digestive System

- Gall Stones
- Diarrhea
- Piles
- Indigestion
- Stomach Ulcers

Diseases of the Respiratory System

- Asthma
- Bronchitis

Diseases of the Heart and Blood Vessels

- Angina
- Correction of Abnormal Heart Rhythms
- Raised Blood Pressure

The Use of Acupuncture in Addiction and Obesity

- Obesity
- Hard Drug Addiction
- Smoking

The Use of Acupuncture in Obstetrics

- Fetal Malposition
- Use of Anesthesia for Labor and Delivery
- Acupuncture Anesthesia

THE ALEXANDER TECHNIQUE

The Alexander Technique is simply a method of channeling ones concentration on how we use our bodies during our daily life activities. This technique was introduced by Frederick Mathias Alexander in the early 19th century. Alexander claimed that there are certain habits that we develop subconsciously which affect our learning, performance and physical functioning. There is a certain inherent posture and position of the body that must not be interfered with; otherwise our bodies lose the capacity of performing to its fullest. The human body is capable of accomplishing greatly complex activities, only when the body is allowed to take its natural course of innate coordination.

One of the methods by which we unconsciously wall off ourselves is referred to as *armoring.* This is a completely unconscious behavior which is most often imbibed in childhood, sometimes even as early as infancy. Although subliminal;, this walling off action often results in feelings of anxiety, loneliness and depression.

It is not difficult to undo this behavior; all one has to do is carefully and closely observe himself. The power of the human mind is such that we can *unlearn* the use of too much tension in our thoughts, movements and relationships, just as easily as we learned them.

The actual treatment is considered as very simple and totally harmless. It is not only guaranteed to achieve a state of agreeableness between mind and body, but it has also shown to be very effective in the complete cure of headaches and backaches. Certain rules of the game are; it is incorrect to stand with round shoulders or slouch; standing too rigid and unbending can again be bad for your spine; the head should be balanced properly above the head and the shoulders should be relaxed and the weight of the body should be *felt* being transferred from one foot to the other while walking. Some more examples of bad posture habits are gripping a pen with all one's might, holding on to the steering wheel too tight. Such habits lead to muscular problems as they involve constant muscle contraction.

To the extent that in many people the head, neck and back are forced out of their regular positions.

The success and authenticity of the Alexander method is endorsed by the fact that when F.M. Alexander *himself* suffered a stroke at the age of 78, he managed to regain use of *all* senses and faculties simply by using this method.

AUTOGENIC TRAINING

This is a less popular technique of alternate medicine. It involves adopting a series of six postures which help the body to relax. It is sort of like yoga. The six exercises can be performed while supine, i.e. lying on one's back, sitting upright in an armchair or sitting on the edge of a chair with head bent forward and chin touching the chest. The focus of the six exercises are 1)respiration and breathing 2)heartbeat, 3)the forehead (to promote a feeling of coolness), 4) the lower abdomen and stomach (for inducing a feeling of warmth), 5) arms and legs (to again induce a feeling of warmth), 6) neck, shoulders, arms and legs, to bring out a feeling of heaviness.

Disorders that are addressed by autogenicity are:

- Irritable Bowel Syndrome
- Digestive disorders
- Muscular aches and cramps
- Ulcers

- Headaches
- High blood pressure
- Anxiety
- Phobias
- Insomnia
- Other psychological illnesses

AYURDVEDIC MEDICINE

This is perhaps the oldest and most well-known methods of medical practice. It is now gaining popularity as an adjuvant therapy alongside orthodox medicine. The working idea behind Ayurvedic medicine is *prevention.*

Methods used for treatment in this field include a variety of herbal medicines, yoga exercises, water and steam baths, massage and a specific diet.

According to the Ayurvedic approach, all things are controlled by three forces, namely *pita, vata* and *kapha.* Pita, synonymous with the sun, is considered to be in control of all body processes, metabolic and functional. Vata, more like the wind, is responsible for the constant smooth working of the brain and nervous system. Kapha, like the moon and its gravitational pull on oceanic tides, is in control of body fluids and the regeneration and growth of various cells in the body. It is believed that a balance of these three forces is essential to good health. Imbalance, resulting due to the excess or deficiency of any one force will result in symptoms of illness.

Another unique approach in Ayurvedic medicine is the categorization of all disorders into four categories:

Mental – covering thoughts and feelings with an emotional trigger, like jealousy, fear, hatred, anger and depression.

Physical- Include mostly all illnesses and disorders

Accidental – Disorders occurring as a result of external trauma

Natural –Disorders and symptoms occurring as a result of the natural progression of age

CHIROPRACTICE

The term chiropractice literally means practice of the hands; it is derived from the Greek words *kheir*, which means hand and *praktikos,* which means practical. The fisrt ever school of chiropractice was established by Daniel Palmer in the late nineteenth century. Palmer was of the opinion that if there were any bones of the body which became displaced somehow, this couldn't affect nervous function.

Chiropractise is most often used for pain relief. It is mostly performed by manipulation of joints and corrects muscle and joint related problems, that is, after a preliminary X-Ray has been performed on the patient. Spinal disorders usually result in a myriad of symptoms all over the body, for example at the hip, leg or arm. Sometimes, manifestations include random symptoms like stress, constipation, asthma and catarrh etc.

People usually seek the help of chiropracticians when they have neck or back pain, or whiplash injuries. People with headaches also seem to be very hopeful towards chiropractise. This is because headaches are associated with rigid neck holding. Other conditions, in which chiropractice has proved its worth, include:

- Tennis elbow
- Pulled muscles
- Injured ligaments and sprains
- Whiplash injury during automobile accident

It has been generally been accepted that chiropractice is an excellent remedy for bone and muscular related issues. However, this is the area it is limited to and does not extend to treatment of more general diseases like high blood pressure and diabetes etc.

CHINESE MEDICINE

Chinese medicine was practiced by Taoist priests of Northern China around 2500 years ago. What they actually practiced was called *Qi Gong* – a sort of meditation which revolved around a certain force which was vital for life. They called this force *qi,* and considered it interwoven with the existence of life. According to them, *qi* was not limited to human life; rather, it was part and parcel all sorts of life in entire universe.

Traditional Chinese medicine was practiced with an intention to *prevent* diseases rather than *cure* them; the focus was to improve the immune system such that it would ward off illnesses and infections.

As mentioned before in, *qi* is a represented in both *yin* (dark, cold and internal) and *yang* (light, warm and external). The ideology of *qi* is that it is manifested in all opposites we experience, for example, night and day, growth and decay, hot and cold. This co-existence of *yin yang* makes them absolutely inseparable. The balance between *yin and yang* being like the successive motion of day and night; at the time of the darkest hour of the night, the cycle has begun to flow smooth and steady towards dawn. At midday, the day starts moving slowly towards the duskiness of night. This pendulous movement is seen in all internal organs of the body, which Chinese herbalist believe to be in in accordance with this diurnal swing of the whole world. The practice of Chinese medicine involves the same meridians and points of energy that are used in acupuncture, as these points are thought to be gateways where *qi* can be blocked or restored.

COLOUR THERAPY

As the name suggests, this faculty of treatment involves the use of colored lights to treat illnesses and restore good health. The different wavelengths of the colors are said to have different effects on different people. The color spectrum is actually a narrow band of wavelengths that can be seen by the human eye. Rays with smaller or larger wavelengths cannot be comprehended by the eye but have a profound effect and function on the entire universe. These are known as electromagnetic radiations and are therefore beneficial to even blind people who cannot see colors.

According to the doctrine of color therapy, everyone human being absorbs electromagnetic radiation from the sun and then emits a unique spectrum of his own. There is a pattern of colors unique to each person. This individual aura of a person can be recorded on film by a technique of photography called Kirlian photography. When a disorder or an illness is present, vibrations from this aura are disturbed and a distorted pattern of colors is obtained.

The spine is the focus of attention of the color therapist as they believe that each vertebra indicates the health of a corresponding part of the body.

Treatment in color therapy, involves the selection of a combination of colors in which the body is bathed completely. The aim is to restore the normal balance of aura specific to that person.

HYDROTHRAPY

Water is used in a number of different ways to either alleviate or completely cure certain ailments. Water has been recognized for its healing powers not only by healers today, but also by Greek, Turkish, European and Chinese civilizations of the past. The famous sauna baths are based on this very principle; hot baths and steam relax the body and relieve muscular stiffness. A cold shower, on the other hand, does just the opposite. It invigorates and refreshes the body. The different effects of these two temperatures is because hot temperature dilates the arteries and veins in skin and stimulate sweating by opening the skin pores, whereas cold water causes constriction of these blood vessels and the blood is redirected towards internal organs. Cold temperatures also cause the skin pores to close.

Water is the new favorite for many physiotherapists today. It is used in the several exercises for people with severe joint and muscle disabilities. In fact, one of the most famous methods of giving birth today is *water birth*. The baby is delivered underwater and comes out swimming.

There are various techniques of treatment within Hydrotherapy. Some of these are:

- Hot baths
- Cold baths
- Neutral baths
- Steam baths
- Sitz baths
- Hot and Cold sprays
- Wrapping
- Cold packs
- Flotation

KINESIOLOGY

This method is involves maintaining good health by ensuring proper function of all muscles. The idea behind this is that each and every muscle is representative of and connected to some specific organ system like the digestive or circulatory system for instance. Therefore, if a muscle is sore, then problems will arise in the related organ system.

The word *kinesis* is Greek in origin and literally means 'motion'. Kinesiology was developed in 1964 by George Goodheart, an American chiropractor. The basis of kinesiology is based on research carried in the early twentieth century, by Dr.Chapman, an osteopath. According to him, there are specific pressure points on the body, which when pressed and massages, allow the free flow of lymph through that region. Kinesiology is said to be particularly effective for people with food allergies and those who are sensitive to certain foods.

MASSAGE

Massage is simply the when a painful part of the body is touched in a way that it is made painless. This is perhaps one of oldest methods of pain relief used by humans. People have found to be using massage therapy in the Far East in 3000 BC. Even in Greece, 5 BC, Hippocrates emphasized upon taking a massage with oil just before a bath.

The basis for today's massage therapy, however, has been laid down by a Swedish fencing master, Per Henrik Ling. He laid the basis for what is known today as the Swedish massage. This deals with soft tissues of the body.

The uses of massage include general relaxation, soothing both mind and body. More specifically, it has been used to treat people having high blood pressure, headaches, sinusitis, insomnia and hyperactive disorders in children. The points of pressure and massage used are again the same as those for acupuncture and Chinese medicine, meridians running along the body related to different organs and organ systems.

REFLEXOLOGY

Reflexology is again an old technique used in ancient times by Egyptians and Chinese civilizations. Reflexology is a special technique whereby certain specific areas of the body are massaged in order to provide relief from pain or other ailments somewhere else in the body. The idea was developed by Dr. William Fitzgerald, an American doctor. He introduced the idea of *zones* and *channels*, along which vital energy flows within the human body. These zones are considered to end in the peripheries of the body, especially the hands and feet. This is why, it is thought, that pain felt in any part of the body can be eased by applying pressure somewhere else, provided it is in the same zone.

The energy flow of the body is said to follow particular routes; it connects every organ and gland in the body and ends in a pressure point on hands and feet, or another peripheral part of the body. Once these routes are disrupted, tenderness arises and indicates that the actual focus of disease is somewhere other than the area which is actually tender. The massage that is performed at points representing the area of disease restores normal flow of energy and heals any damage that may have occurred.

Areas where reflexology has proved to be effective include

- Back pain, headache and toothache
- Digestive diseases
- Stress and Tension
- Influenza and colds
- Asthma
- Arthritis

An important point to note while seeking the help of Reflexologists is that there are certain conditions in which the use of reflexology should be avoided, in fact it may even be harmful. These are:

- Diabetes
- Certain heart disorders
- Osteoporosis
- Thyroid gland disorders
- Phlebitis (inflammation of veins)
- Pregnancy
- Arthritis of the feet

REIKI

Reiki is a Japanese complementary therapy of alternate medicine which revolves around *universal life energy*. This philosophy was developed by a Japanese theologist, Dr. Mikao Usui. He developed this ability of transferring reiki energy after a long period of meditation. Eventually Dr. Usui was able to help people by transferring this energy.

In order to benefit from Reiki, one has to be *initiated* to reiki energy by a reiki master. Reiki energy is considered the most effective form of life energy and has the maximum vibration of all energies. Once a person takes a session of reiki, they allow reiki energy to be taken up by their bodies. It is in effect a subconscious decision: how much reiki energy to absorb.

The instruments of healing in reiki are ones *hands*. Reiki is performed by placing hands over the area of interest. The person undergoing the reiki session may experience feelings of attraction, repulsion, flow, heat, cold and tingling, reflecting the response of their bodies to the session of reiki.

It can be safely concluded that reiki is a method of healing that can be made available anywhere and to anyone. It helps one achieve a more relaxed approach in life.

SHIATSU

The origin of shiatsu can be dated back to 2000 years ago in China. It has been influenced by the Japanese and East and West civilizations before it took its form today. The Eastern ideology of *ki, chi,* and *prana* energy that exists in the universe and flows through certain channels in the human body stands true here as well.

As in acupuncture, there are points representative of these energy flow tracts and are referred to as *tsubos.*

Applications of shiatsu include treatment of insomnia, anxiety, headaches and back pain. It is believed that the giver and receiver of shiatsu, both benefit physically and spiritually from this energy transfer.

There are believed to be several auras or layers of energy which surround the human body. These are the etheric body, astral body, mental body, causal body and soul or higher self. It is believed that as a person grows physically and mentally, different auras come into use and energy is passed on from one layer to another.

Another belief in the practice of Shiatsu is the existence of seven centres of energy, known as *chakras*. These are situated along the midline of the body and are positioned on a spiritual spiral, the *sushumna*, which travels down the body from head to toe. The *chakras* are:

- Crown chakra
- Brow or forehead chakra
- Throat chakra
- Heart chakra
- Personality chakra
- Sexual chakra
- Root chakra

Each chakra is representative of certain areas and functions of the body.

AROMATHERAPY

Aromatherapy is a practice of healing that involves the use of concentrated oils which give off a very strong aroma and are extracted from plants. All plants have different odors due to the presence of different essential oils present within. These oils may be present in the stem, leaves, root, bark, fruit or seeds of the plant.

Archaeologists have found several references to the art of healing by using plant essences in art and writings belonging to Egyptian, Chinese and Persian civilisations.

Although proper research is lacking in the field, the mode of action of aromatherapy is that individual essential oils have antiseptic, antibiotic, sedative and tonic properties which align themselves with the body's natural defense systems. Common ailments and the essential oils they benefit from are mentioned below:

- Anxiety- *basil, bergamot, geranium, lavender, melissa, neroli*
- Depression- *bergamot, chamomile, peppermint, rosemary*

- Fatigue- *clary sage, eucalyptus, juniper berry, peppermint, rosemary.*
- Dry skin- *bergamot, chamomile, geranium, jasmine, lavender, melissa, neroli*
- Oily skin- *cypress, lemon, tea tree*
- Acne- *bergamot, cedarwood, chamomile, cypress, eucalyptus, fennel, geranium, juniper berry, lavender, lemon, myrhh, parsley, rose*
- Eczcma – *chamomile, geranium, juniper berry, lavender, melissa*
- Amenorrhea- *chamomile, clary sage, fennel, geranium, safe*
- Dysmenorrhea- *cypress, geranium, rose*
- Hot flushes- *chamomile, jasmine, lavender, petitgrain*
- Mastitis- *chamomile, clary sage, geranium, lavender, rose*
- Period pain- *lavender, marjoram, clary sage*

HOMEOPATHY

Homeopathy aims to treat the person as a whole rather than concentrate on one specific symptom or set of symptoms. Even details such as the emotional and psychological wellbeing of the person are taken into consideration when prescribing a homeopathy medicine. The idea behind this approach is that disease is a loss of balance within the body.

A homeopathy medicine must be suitable not only for the symptoms of a person but also to his temperament and to his character.

The working concept here is that 'like cures like'. This is actually a primordial concept that was originated by Hippocrates back in 5th century BC. Long afterwards, a German doctor, Dr. Samuel Hahnemann was captivated by this theory and started conducting research on it. He found that the extract of the cinchona bark, a treatment for malaria, produces the exact symptoms of malaria when a healthy person ingested it in small quantities. He was convinced that this response of the body was actually a defense mechanism of the body. Therefore, he concluded, that this minute dose could be used to fight the disease in someone who actually had malaria. This is what encouraged conducting further trials, most of which were successful.

The basis of modern homeopathy is the research and hard work of Hahnemann. The medicines used in today's homeopathy practice are plant, mineral and animal extracts and are used in extremely small amounts. Substances which are used in this method of alternate medicine are initially soaked in alcohol so as to extract their essential components. The resulting solution is referred to as *mother tincture* and is then diluted continuously by factors of ten or hundred. Each dilution is shaken vigorously after dilution and this is thought to potentiate and energize the medicine. These solutions are then made into either tablets, solutions, ointments, powders or suppositories etc. High potency treatments are used for stronger symptoms and the lower potency ones are used for milder symptoms.

Today, homeopathy has reached the stage where it is recognized by allopathic doctors and is, in fact, even resorted to in certain medical conditions.

PREPARATION OF THE POTIONS

Now that we have discussed what the properties of medicinal herbs are and how they interact with human biology, we need to learn how to prepare them such that their benefits are maximized. To begin with, if you are starting to practice herbal medicine on a small scale you will have to grow your herbs. This is probably one of the most pleasurable aspects of becoming a herbalist.

You know very well that plants are living creatures much like us, they require a specific sort of attention and care which is essential to their development, much like nurturing a child. It is believed that plants have a subtle healing energy of force which they store and transmit to an ill person when required. This is why herbalists avoid the use of iron implements to cut herbs; iron Is said to destroy this energy.

The *time* when you start growing herbs or cutting them, is also a factor which affects the healing properties of plants. Medicinal properties of plants are affected by the moon, seasons and even different times of the day. St. John's wort is called so because the best time to gather this plant is said to be around the time of St. John's day, which is around midsummer's day. This is practical advice, because this is the time that this plant comes to flower!

Certain French traditions state that herbs and flowers should never be collected at the time of full moon because the moon absorbs their energy and strength. Roots, however must be collected at exactly this time of the month, as they are said to be extremely potent at full moon.

Scientists have seconded herbalists here, and have proved these 'superstitions' to be point on and in accordance with diurnal biorhythms of plants and animals. Research has proven that the content of morphine in the opium plant is higher at 11 a.m. than at 3 p.m., also the morphine content is greatest till three weeks after the plant has flowered.

Another example is the rhubarb root, come winter the laxative effect of this herb is lost because of the near nil concentration of anthraquinone, however, wait till summer and the anthraquinone levels shoot up again. Certain pointers for collecting herbs are listed below:

- Gather leaves just when the flowers about to open
- Flowers should be picked just before they are in full bloom
- Underground parts of a plant must be collected when the rest of the plant is dry and dead
- Bark is best after a bout of rain because it is damp and easily separated from the tree

- Gums and resins should be collected after dry, hot weather
- Roots and rhizomes need a good shake to get out of the soil
- Don't over-pick any area; leave enough to propagate for next year
- Collect plants away from industrial areas; the lead, chemicals, herbicides, insecticides and pesticides deplete all medicinal qualities of plants
- Store herbs in a paper bag or a wicker basket; *never* use plastic bags
- If the weather is warm, spread the plants out to dry before they start fermenting; avoid direct sunlight because this will release and disperse all essential oils
- Storage should be in a dark, cool place, either in paper bags, cardboard boxes or air-tight glass bottles.
- Aerial parts of plants must be discarded after one year
- Bark and roots can be used up to two years.

Coming to the prescription of drugs, it is *as* important as the herbs being used. Different methods or preparing the same herb helps extract different ingredients.

Infusions

These are prepared by pouring boiling water over fresh or dried herbs. The best solvent for gums, mucilages, tannins and saponins is water, preferably spring water as it is less hard than tap water. Water isn't very good at dissolving oils because of the hydrophobic nature of oils. The infusion cup or pot should be covered so as to prevent escape of volatile oils. Take 30 gm of the herb with 500 ml water, and drink after infusing for a minimum of fifteen minutes.

Decoctions

These are made by boiling hard parts of plants like the roots and barks in water. Those containing volatile oils should only be boiled for a short while and left in the water as they cool. Containers used for boiling must always be either of enamel, reinforced glass or stainless-steel, *never* use aluminum utensils, they leave traces of aluminum in the herbs. Use 600 ml water for 30 gm of root or bark. Simmer for twenty minutes once it boils.

Tinctures

These are made by macerating herbs in a mixture of alcohol and water for at least two weeks, this helps extract medicinal properties of the plant. The alcohol is an excellent solvent for the extraction of oils, gums and resins. The alcohol also acts as a preservative. Another method of preparing tinctures is by percolation; the powdered herb is subject to a constant flow of alcohol and water which is collected at the floor of the percolation chamber.

The most appropriate amount for tincture is 200 gm of herb in one litre of alcohol and water. The strength of alcohol varies with the nature of the substance that has to be extracted from the herb. It can be as dilute as a twenty five percent fortified alcohol and as strong as a ninety percent Polish vodka.

Glycerol

This is an excellent option for preserving an extract which is aqueous in nature. Substances like marshmallow, comfrey and mucilaginous roots are easily preserved in it. Take 200 gm of the herb and place it in a saucepan. Add one liter of water and boil until 600 ml is left, leave the root to macerate for four hours before straining and pressing. Now add 400 ml of glycerol and use it the same way you would use a tincture.

Fluid extracts

These are liquid extracts and are of very high concentration such that one part volume of the extract is one part by weight of the herb. Therefore, one litre fluid extract contains one kilogram of herb. The active ingredient is extracted by alcohol which is evaporated off, leaving behind the solid extract; this is then dissolved in dilute alcohol according to the required strength.

Syrups

These are not recommended for people with diabetes. Honey is preferred over sugar. It is ideal because of its antibiotic and expectorant qualities. This is the best preparation of a cough syrup. Syrups are made by decocting herbs in one liter of water and straining it after it has cooled. Then, a quarter of its weight of honey is added. The liquid is heated gently until it becomes more viscous. Flavoring agents like mint or aniseed can be added to make syrups more palatable.

Powders

Herbs can easily be powdered by using a coffee grinder. These powders can then be mixed with honey to make an electuary, or they can be put into gelatin capsules. These should be avoided by people who have a weak digestive system.

Pills

This is the easiest way to take medicine, which is why pharmaceuticals today manufacture medicines mostly in this form. Coarsely grounded herbs can be rolled into dough with slippery elm powder. Once dry this can be cut into small pills.

Baths

Herbal baths are exactly as luxurious as they sound. The hot herbal water opens up the skin pores and helps with absorption of the herbal extracts into the body. Make 4 liters of a decoction and strain before mixing it into the bath. Alternatively, a muslin bag filled with herbs can be kept under the tap water so the water runs through it. Herbal baths are recommended for treating unruly children or babies around teething time, especially bathing with chamomile or limeflower extract can work magic. A simple herbal bath can be made by adding five to six drops of an essential oil in the bath. Lavender is best for relaxation, pine oil for muscle aches and cramps and rosemary is excellent for uplifting a bad mood.

Ointments

Ointments are an ingenious method of ensuring long term contact of healing herbs with the affected area. When making ointments, one must be careful of the composition. If it becomes too greasy it seals in heat, and this can have an adverse effect in certain conditions.

An easy way of making an ointment is from chickweed, sunflower iol and beeswax. Take 300 gm of the chickweed and immerse it in 480 ml of sunflower oil. Boil in a double boiler. Bring the water in the outer boiler to boil and then leave it to simmer on mild heat for three to four hours. The chickweed should lose its color by the end of this. Strain the oil afterwards and heat it again. Add 60 gm beeswax and heat till the beeswax has melted. You may add a few drops of lavender for fragrance, and a drop of tincture or benzoin for every 30 ml of oil, in order to preserve it.

Poultices

Poultices are applied while hot in order to relieve inflammation and help improve blood circulation. The heat hence allows more oxygen to reach the wound and this helps get rid of bacteria. Poultices can be made from bread or common vegetables. Carrots for example, make an excellent poultice; boil carrots until they are soft and then mash them up to a pulp. Add some olive oil and spread out the carrot mix on a double layer of cotton gauze. They leave this atop a sieve on boiling water; the steam should be able to permeate it easily.

Compresses

Compresses allow the application of an infusion or a decoction directly to skin. A compress can be made by soaking a cloth in a hot decoction, wringing out the fluid quickly and placing on the skin. It is preferable to use two cloths alternatively.

Plasters

These are a very useful method of local treatment for muscular and rheumatic pains. They are also effective for healing broken skin and tissues. The active herbal substances and melted in beeswax and spread on linen which is then plastered on to skin. The heat of the body helps keep the wax soft and also promoted absorption of the herb.

DISPOSABLE INDISPOSITIONS AND THEIR HERBAL TREATMENTS

Herbal medicine is nature's gift to living beings. Even animals have an instinctive affinity for certain curative herbs when are developing an illness. One can only be convinced of the healing power of these herbs when one uses them and subsequently benefits. Not only are these natural substances extremely effective; they cost a fraction of what over-the-counter medicines do. The irony is that most over-the-counter medicines use herbal extracts as their active ingredients.

Perhaps the best part of herbal medicine is that one can grow these herbs easily at home. Even though we always criticize grandparents and their vast knowledge of home remedies, it is these remedies that are most useful. Although modern medicine has advanced to levels unfathomable by the human mind, people still prefer herbal medicine over it.

Although one can use herbal remedies for common ailments without a second thought, the one danger of self-medication with herbs is that one put's off going to a professional doctor and resorts to at-home herbal treatment even for the more morbid diseases. If you are unsure about what medicine to take, or if your symptoms persist for more than two days then it is imperative that you consult a professional.

Here are some common illnesses and their herbal remedies.

Common cold

The common cold is so *common* because the causative agents, i.e. viruses, are ever changing in their genetic structure. This is why scientists have yet not managed to develop a medicine or vaccine against them. Also, viruses are activated when they are taken up by the cells of the body and this is precisely why it difficult to destroy them. The only way this illness can be contained is by strengthening the body's immune system.

At the first signs of an oncoming cold, you must take this concoction:

- Fresh root of ginger, sliced, 30 gm
- Cinnamon sticks, broken into little pieces, 1-2
- Coriander seeds, 2.5 gm
- Cloves, 4
- Water, 600 ml

Put all ingredients in a pan and bring to a boil. Once boiled, cover the pan and leave it to simmer for 20 minutes. Just before turning off the heat, add a slice of lemon. Strain the solution and add honey to sweeten slightly. Drink one cup while hot, every couple of hours.

Another effective remedy is a herbal tea, constituting equal parts of:

- Hyssop, 30 gm
- Elderflowers, 30 gm
- Mint leaves, 30 gm

Pour 500 ml of boiling water onto this mixture and cover (to prevent evaporation of essential oils), let it stand for 10-15 minutes. Strain and drink one cup every two, three hours.

Finally, something which may sound peculiar but is useful is, a mustard foot bath:

- Mustard powder, 1 tablespoon
- Hot water, 1 litre

Bathe both feet for about 8-10 minutes, just before bedtime.

Apart from this, you must eat foods rich in vitamin C as this boosts the immune system. In order to load up on vitamin C, you must eat lots of oranges, rose-hip tea, and lemon and honey tea. Apart from this, garlic, green onion and common onion must be taken in moderate quantities, but *raw.* Other helpful foods include watercress, cabbage, black pepper and mustard.

Catarrh

Catarrh is common accomplice of the common cold. The best treatment fior this is inhalation of steam. The steam can be made more effective by the addition of volatile aromatic oils. These preparations can be made by pouring boiling water over herbs or oils and immediately covering with a towel or a thick cloth. It should be large enough to allow your head to fit inside and yet still seal off corners, to prevent the steam from escaping. This treatment is more aptly called aromatherapy, and is one of the mainstream treatments of herbal medicine. The preparation is as:

- Eucalyptus, 3 drops
- Peppermint, 3 drops
- Pine, 3 drops
- Wintergreen, 3 drops

Add 10 ml benzoin tincture to this mix. Boil 500 ml water, wait for about a minute and then pour it in the bowl. An alternative method is to put this mixture of essential oils and tincture into a simple vaporizer. This should be done at night so that the vapors filling the bedroom are inhaled throughout the night.

Catarrh is worsened by mucus forming foods like eggs, milk and other dairy products. Mushrooms must also be avoided in this condition. Instead, you must eat lots of fruits and drink herbal mint or thyme tea. Other helpful herbs include garlic, onions, oregano, cayenne pepper and ginger. These can be added while cooking.

Sore throat

A sore throat is a sore pain. The only way to ease this pain is to gargle it out.

- Sage leaves, fresh or dried, 1 handful
- Apple cider vinegar, 1/2 tablespoon
- Water, 500 ml

Boil water and pour over the sage leaves, cover immediately. Once it has cooled, add the vinegar. Gargle with this solution every four hours.

A more 'professional' mixture can be made by purchasing the following tinctures:

- Golden seal *(Hydrastis Canadensis)*, 5ml
- Balm of gilead (*populous gileadensis)*, 5 ml
- Myrrh (*Commiphora molmol)* 5 ml
- Liquorice (*Glycyrrhiza glabra*) 5 ml
- Oil of cinnamon, 4 drops

Add water to increase amount to 200 ml. Shake this mixture well and use only a teaspoon in a warm cup of water for gargling.

If the sore throat persists, then it means a bacterial infection has superseded the viral infection, and now appropriate antibiotics should be soughted.

Coughs

A persistent cold eventually results in infection of the deeper respiratory passages and this manifests as cough. The cough is actually a reflex, when it comes in contact with an irritant, which is most likely harmful for the body, it expels it out with high pressure. This is the same working principle of a sneeze. Coughing also helps move up the layer of mucus in our throat and nasal passages which contain dust particles and trap bacteria. This process of expectoration can be boosted by simple kitchen remedies:

- Large onion, sliced into rings, 1
- Honey, enough to cover all onion rings

Leave the onions and honey overnight in a deep bowl. The onion juice is then strained, mixing the onion juice and honey. This concoction is to be taken by the teaspoonful, every couple of hours.

Another general cough remedy includes:

- 2 woody liquorice sticks (*Glycyrrhiza glabra*)
- Root of Marshmallow (*Althaea officinalis*) 8 gm
- Wild bark (*Prunus serotina*) 8 gm
- Coltsfoot flowers (*Tussilago farfara*) 8 gm
- Borage leaves and flowers (*Borago offinalis*) 8 gm
- Hyssop (*Hyssopus officinalis*) 8 gm
- Linseed (*Linum usitatissimum*) 30 gm
- Lemon, ½

Pour about 1 ¼ liters of water onto these components, stir and cover. Let it stand. Then after one hour, heat it again and strain. Pour in some honey, and drink one cup every two hours.

It is an age old remedy to rub a mixture of oil of camphor and vegetable oil on the chest. This helps relieve cough. Again, mucus forming foods like dairy products must be avoided and the use of garlic, onion, ginger, cabbage and almonds must be increased.

One important point to note is that if the cough persists for more than a few days then a serious underlying disease is more likely.

Indigestion

An occasional episode of indigestion is normal. However, when it occurs on a regular basis then there is something amiss either in the *type* of food being eaten or in the dietary *habits.* The simple and most effective treatment for indigestion is to change ones diet. One of the biggest mistakes people make today is to take scores of antacids in order to neutralize the stomach acid. While this is effective immediately, it actually has the reverse effect in the long run, as the acid producing cells then produce even more acid. One of the most effective antacid herbal medicine treatments include a herbal tea consisting of:

- Gentian root *(Gentiana lutea)* 8 gm
- Angelica root *(Angelica archangelica)* 8 gm
- Anise *(Pimpinella anisum)* 15 gm
- Peppermint (*Mentha piperita*) 15 gm
- Chamomile *(Matricaria chamomilla)* 15 gm
- Dried mandarin peel *(Citrus reticulata)* 4 pieces
- Liquorice *(Glycyrrhiza glabra)* 1 stick, broken and grinded

Add liquorice, gentian and angelica root in a litre of water and boil it. Let it simmer for ten minutes. Remove from heat and add the rest of the ingredients. Cover it and let it stand for about twenty minutes. Strain and drink one cup after a routine meal.

Diarrhea

Acute diarrhea is a reflex of the digestive system to expel toxins or harmful substances just a couple of hours after they are taken into the body. This may be a sign or serious disease. Especially if diarrhea occurs persistently for more than two days, then one must look for a professional.

Once diarrhea ensues in children one must become extra cautious because children can get dehydrated very quickly, this can lead to electrolyte imbalance which eventually has serious consequences.

Toxins ingested into the stomach can be neutralized by taking in pectin, tannins and garlic. The pectin is an absorbent and tannin has astringent properties, both of these help restore normal bowel action. Garlic is a potent antibiotic and can be used to negate the bacterial activity.

Diarrhea can be controlled by

- Tormentil (*Potentilla tormentilla*) 30 gm
- Cinnamon, 1 stick
- Caraway seeds, 1 teaspoon
- Ginger, 2 slices

Add all substances to 600 ml water, boil and leave to simmer for fifteen minutes. Strain and drink one cup four to five times a day.

Another herb relevant in diarrhea is the rhubarb root (*Rheum officinale*), interestingly it's effect varied with the concentration ingested. When taken in large doses, rhubarb functions as a laxative, whereas when it is taken in small amounts of less than a gram, then it is an effective antidiarrheal. An easy preparation is to mix powder of rhubarb root with honey and fill it in a size 00 capsule. This must be taken three times a day.

Once the acute incident of diarrhea is controlled, another elixir must be taken:

- Arrowroot powder (*Maranta arundinaceae*) 8 gm
- Slippery elm powder (*Ulmus fulva*) 8 gm
- Cinnamon powder, 1 pinch

Mix together all three of these; take a teaspoon of the mixture and mix into a small amount of plain yoghurt. This should be taken several times throughout the day.

The electrolyte misbalance that occurs due to diarrhea can be corrected by taking some warm water with honey.

High blood sugar

This is a sure sign of diabetes. It can occur either to ineffective insulin production or due to insufficient response of tissues to insulin. Controlling the level of sugar in blood is absolutely essential in the initial stages as there are fatal consequences of high blood sugar level.

Cinnamon is very effective in reducing the sugar level. It can be taken in a variety of ways; cinnamon tea, raw cinnamon powder or simply sprinkled over food. Cinnamon tea can be made as follows:

- Cinnamon powder, ½ teaspoon
- Water 500 ml

Wrap the cinnamon powder in a muslin cloth and boil with water, let it simmer for 10 minutes. Cover the mixture after turning off the heat. Drink three times daily and check sugar levels after one week.

High cholesterol and heart health

High cholesterol is a danger sign as it predisposes to heart attacks and strokes. Just like high blood sugar, maintaining low cholesterol is essential to maintaining good health. Certain herbs known to reduce the levels of cholesterol, and therefore the risk of heart disease include garlic, cloves and fenugreek seeds. These can be taken raw or slightly cooked both.

Urinary tract infections

Urinary tract infections are more common in women, this is because women have a shorter urinary tract than men and there are more chances of disease causing bacteria to ascend to the bladder and cause infection. Signs of urinary tract infection include painful urination, an urge to urinate as soon as possible and poor control over urine flow. A very effective remedy for this is cranberry juice, which contains substances which prevent the bacteria from attaching to the bladder wall and hence promote their removal from the body.

Cranberry juice can be taken as it is, cranberries can be eaten as a whole or the extract of cranberries can be used to make tea This should be taken daily until symptoms of the infection resolve.

Joint pain and arthritis

Joint pains are a result of arthritis which is inflammation of the joints. This can be due to age related wear out of joints or it can be due to a more serious condition in which the body produces antibodies against its own tissues, especially small joints. An efficacious herb for curing joint pains is turmeric. The active component of turmeric, i.e. curcumin, is well known for its anti-inflammatory properties. Turmeric can easily be taken with soup, sauces and vegetables and other food substances.

Cancer prevention

Cancer is one of the most fatal diseases of the twentieth century. It occurs because of mutations which occur within cellular DNA. These mutations occur due to exposure to radiation and other environmental hazards. Normally the cell has anti-oxidants which reverse these mutations or prevent them from occurring in the first place. However, these anti-oxidants are not always sufficient. Therefore, several herbs with anti-oxidant properties have been identified. These include cinnamon, cloves, oregano, green tea, turmeric and garlic. These herbs are known to kill or inhibit growth or cancer cells.

PRINCIPLES OF HERBAL MEDICINE

As we have discussed previously, herbal medicine is not limited to or derived from a single region. It has been modified by several successive civilizations. Therefore, if you analyze the different ideologies ruling over most methods of alternate medicine, you will find that the core idea behind each healing method is actually a conglomeration of eastern wisdom and eastern ideologies.

The principles of herbal medicine, which form the basis of its practice, can broadly be divided into eastern and western philosophies.

The Eastern Point of View

The age old symbol of yin and yang are as representative of traditional Chinese medicine as the serpent is of conventional medicine. This is the basis for all medical practice in the eastern world. The general notion is that *everything* in the universe is born from and associated with the yin and yang. These two opposing forces are as mutually exclusive as they are interdependent. It's easy to identify with this theory as there is an opposite for everything in the universe; even Newton's law of 'equal and opposite reaction' somewhat endorses this idea.

The Chinese believe that just like yin and yang cause a successive fluctuation in the universe, they are also responsible for maintaining balance within the human body. An imbalance due to excess or deficiency of either force can lead to disease or illness.

Within the context of yin and yang, the body is said to consist of several energy pathways, the most important of which is Qi, pronounced 'chi'. It is believed that Qi is the energy which enables us to think, feel and move. It's considered as the power engine of the soul. The pathways of Qi are basically channels, more appropriately called *meridians*, which travel throughout the body and are connected to at least one organ or organ systems. There are twelve such meridians within the body and this is where Qi flows through and maintains healthy organ function. However, any degree of physical, emotional and environmental insult can cause a blockade to the flow of this energy, consequently resulting in illness.

Traditional Chinese herbal medicine sees the human body, mind and soul as one package that needs an upgrade as a whole. This differs from the western philosophy of separating out a single issue and solely addressing it.

Certain theories which act as pillars for the function of herbal medicine include:

The Five Element Theory

These five elements are wood, fire, earth, metal and water; they are said to be part and parcel of human beings and their natural biology. The five elements are believed to be representative of the different seasons as well as different organs in the body. The associations are as follow:

- **Wood**: *Season-* Spring, *Organs-* Liver and Gallbladder
- **Fire**: *Season-*Early Summer, *Organs-* Heart and Small intestines
- **Earth**: *Season-*Late Summer, *Organs-* Stomach and Spleen
- **Metal**: *Season-* Autumn, *Organs-* Lungs and Large Intestines
- **Water**: *Season-*Winter, *Organs-* Kidneys and Bladder

Another ideology of eastern herbal medicine is that, in contrast to the western idea of mind and body being completely different entities, eastern medicine believes each organ entity is a one complete system of mind, body and soul. This is why Chinese herbalists believe that the liver is the organ which 'plans' and 'stores anger', whereas the gall bladder is the 'decision-making' organ.

Before treating their patients, eastern herbalists ask a series of questions related to work, lifestyle and nature of the person so that they can classify the personality of the person according of the five elements. It is intriguing to know that according to the Chinese, all elements are present in everyone, with varying aspects at different times.

A complimentary set of principles that the Chinese use are the *Eight Guiding Principles*. These principles are used to determine the balance or imbalance of energetic forces within the body, as well as the nature of the illness that is being experienced. The eight guiding principles are four diametric fundamentals:

- **Cold/ Heat**

This is used to ascertain the level or energy of the patient; if it's cold, the patient will be said to have a slow metabolism, pale skin and mild fever. A hot predisposition, however, will classify on as having a high metabolic rate, increased heat sensation in the body, high grade fever and red, flushed skin.

- **Interior/ Exterior**

This is a simple classification based on the nature of disease. For instance, interior conditions are those where the pathogens enter organs, deep vessels and nerves, bones, brain and spinal cord. The exterior conditions, on the contrary, are those affecting the periphery of the body, like the hair, muscles, joints, skin, blood vessel and nerves.

- **Deficiency/ Excess**

This is a measure of the potency of an illness. Eastern herbalists view a 'deficient' state as one where the patient lacks blood, energy, heat and/or fluids. A classic example of a deficient state is chronic illness. When the status quo is more towards excess, the body is considered to have too much of either blood or energy. An acute condition would fall in this category.

- **Yin/Yang**

The interdependent opposing forces of life, also a fair summary of the above mentioned rules; yin represents the fairer, feminine, chronic and cold energy which is associated with solid organs. Yang, on the other hand, is the acute, masculine counterpart with an emanation of heat and representation of the more hollow organs. Both are necessary for good health and are considered to be present in balanced amounts in all organisms.

These are the foundation principles on which eastern medicine bases its prescription and healing properties on. A combination of these principles, determines the exact nature of three components of the body: energy, moisture and blood.

The Western Point of View

According to western herbalists, different drugs have different effects on different parts of the body because the body is composed of isolated molecules itself. A herb is considered to constitute of a combination of subtle chemicals which are gentle and dilute in action. The drug action is not restricted to a single specific site, rather it affects different tissues with different functions; this action of drugs has a synergistic effect throughout the body.

Western herbalists are now shifting away from their ideology of molecular disturbances and moving towards a holistic approach where an imbalance is considered to occur in the whole body. Thus, modern herbal medicine is reviving traditional concepts of synergistic patterns of behavior of organs.

In the holistic practice of herbal medicine, certain concepts need to be clarified. According to western healers, there are three major principles which are important in the practice of alternate medicine:

1) a herb's affinity for a disease with a specific pattern,

2) a herb's affinity for an organ or organ system, and

3) a herb's affinity for natural inclination of self-governance in the person

PATTERN AND ENERGY OF A DISEASE

According to Aristotle, there are four main qualities of the natural world: *dry, damp, hot* and *cold.* These ideas were used in Greek medicine and very aptly described the fundamental patterns and properties of plants. Henceforth, from damp to dry or hot to cold, Greek healers were able to treat a specific disease. Cayenne, for example, is a warm, stimulating herb; it improves circulation of the blood and also helps the heart pump blood more efficiently. Lavender is another drug with quite the opposite effects. It has an overall cooling effect, and prevents headaches by slowing blood supply, and hence heat, to the head. A moist choice to counter dry mucous membranes and dry coughs. In conditions where there is excessive secretion such as diarrhea, then blackberry leaves, which have astringent effects, are very helpful in drying out the secretions.

Although Aristotle's philosophy was widely accepted, there were certain notions put forward by conventional physicians at the time, which were incorporated into Aristotle's theory, altogether achieving a new set of principles. The two basic conditions identified by conventional physicians are *status strictus,* i.e. too much tension and *status laxus* i.e. too much relaxation.

These two conditions, along with the four qualities identified by Aristotle, amounts to a system of six kinds which are representative of six states which have been recognized by physicians of the early twentieth century, Therefore the six conditions which western herbalists identify with are:

- **Heat / Excitation**

As the name suggests, this state identifies with all symptoms of inflammation. One of the five core qualities of inflammation is *calor*, i.e. heat. Other symptoms of inflammation, redness, swelling and pain are also part and parcel of this condition. The general concept of 'excitability' refers to an excess of stimulation leading to oversensitive nerves and an overactive immune system. The heat somewhat serves as a catalyst for oxidizing reactions within the body. The only way to oppose them or slow them down is by taking cool refreshments, especially those made with fruits and berries. The contrasting action of these drinks is now commonly referred to as *antioxidant.*

Certain cooling remedies include peach, hawthorn, rose, lime, lemon, rhubarb, yellow dock root, elder and honeysuckle,

- **Wind / Constriction**

This is where the 'constricting' concept of western herbalists comes in. it relates to constriction or tension; symptoms which are representative of this condition include sudden unforeseen changes or onsets or volatile symptoms, usually involving a feeling of restlessness of body and soul. The pulse is said to be hard and 'resistant'. Although the main system involved in this case is the nervous system, the skin and blood vessels may also be involved as they can cause similar 'constriction' symptoms by blocking skin pores, blood flow or other fluids. The patient may feel feverish and fails to perspire normally. The treatment here is use of herbs which are diaphoretics, relaxants and antispasmodics. Herbs possessing these qualities include catnip, hops, valerian, wild lettuce, vibernum, blue vervain, lobelia and, the most effective, agrimony. These are very bitter tasting substances owing to their astringent activity.

- **Dry / Atrophy**

As with most living creatures, seventy percent of the human body is made of water. This constitution is essential because water is responsible for absorption and distribution of nutrient to all cells of the body. In case of dryness, there will be an overall negative effect on every system of the body. The symptoms of dryness are very obvious: a dry tongue, lack-luster and sunken eyes, constipation, dry flaky skin. If the condition is severe then weight loss and weakness may also occur. The pulse if felt as weak and feeble. The treatment here consists of lots of fluids, both water and oil. Therefore herbs which stimulate release of fluids are recommended in this case. Bitters are an excellent option as they stimulate salivation. Other applicable herbs include Marshmallow, fenugreek, cleavers, slippery elm, plantain, comfrey, ginseng, mushrooms, nettles, psyllium seeds, sage and angelica.

- **Damp / Relaxation**

The tissues are very relaxed in this situation and are damp because they have open pores which encourage the loss of fluids. The fluids are said to overflow out of the body tissues and this cause them to sag. Symptoms are related to excess loss of fluid in the form of menses, urine, sweat, sputum and diarrhea. The loss of body fluids leads to a resultant loss of essential electrolytes. The patient may complain of hemorrhoids, prolapsed uterus or hemorrhoids. The pulse is relaxed but the patient is usually pale. These people also need herbs rich in astringents; these include bayberry bark, alum root, raspberry lead, sumach, blackberry, oak bark and nettles.

- **Damp / Stagnation**

Although this sounds similar to a previously mentioned condition, it is slightly different because the fluids, although free flowing, are not lost to the environment; rather they build up and are retained in the body tissues. This fluid retention results in the precipitation of mucopolysaccharides. These are sticky, viscous substances which tend to slow down internal processes. Some people also consider this accumulation of fluid as toxic blood. In a way this theory makes sense because the liver is unable to carry out its detoxifying functions and these harmful substances accumulate in the body causing skin outbreaks. The thyroid also slows down and results in a low metabolic rate. This situation requires a massive cleanup with purifiers like red clover, Oregon grape root, dandelion, black walnut, burdock and yellow dock root, as well as cleansing laxatives like rhubarb, butternut and cascara. The thyroid can be speeded up by taking hulls of black walnut, after blackening them

- **Cold / Depression**

This is a condition which is very much the opposite of the heat and excitation. There is an internal slowness or cold as herbalists describe it that is very different from the chill of external cold. The skin is cold, dull, pale and almost blue-black because of thickened blood. The body activities have been slowed down because the body cells co-exist with foreign bacteria, viruses or parasites which consume all nutrients, leaving the other cells to starve. Also these foreign organisms release toxins which have harmful effects of the body. There is a genera predisposition to necrosis, sepsis and putrefaction; the pulse is weak; the tongue is dark and the person is depressed. Useful remedies are stimulating and warming herbs like rosemary, angelica, thyme, sage, cayenne, mustard, cabbage, echinacea, sassafras and prickly ash. Astringent and laxative substances have also successfully cured such disorders.

These are the principles and lines of thought which the herbalist is working on which he prescribes medicine to his patients. The eastern and western theories have combines to formulate unmatchable criteria for the diagnosis and treatment of diseases.

HERB ACTIONS

The attributes and features of herbs are absolutely unparalleled. Similarly, their modes of actions are also very distinctive and diverse. To the extent, that, certain terms have been coined *specifically* to describe the actions of these herbs. The understanding of these terms is imperative to the understanding of and the use of different herbs. These terms and their implications are mentioned below:

Alterative	A term given to a substance which speeds up tissue renewal and enables more efficient functioning
Anodyne	One that soothes and eases pain
Antihelminthic	A drug that cause the death & therefore elimination of parasites
Antiperiodic	One that prevents recurring diseases from happening. E.g. Malaria
Antiscorbutic	A substance rich in vitamin C and hence preventing scurvy
Antiseptic	Substance applied to wounds and infections because it inhibits growth of bacteria and eventually eliminates them
Antispasmodic	One that diminishes muscle spasms
Aperient	A medicine enabling natural bowel movement
Aphrodisiac	A substance which stimulates the sexual organs and arouses sexual

	desire
Aromatic	One that gives off a strong aroma/fragrance
Astringent	A substance causing the contraction of cells; eventually causing contraction of blood vessels and tissues
Balsamic	A drug used for colds and abrasions; contains resins and benzoic acid
Bitter	A substance bitter in taste and helpful in stimulating appetite
Cardiac	Compounds which have a direct and profound effect on the heart
Carminative	A preparation used for providing relief from flatulence and abdominal griping pains
Cathartic	A substance causes expulsion of bowel contents and easing defecation
Cholagogue	A compound stimulating the release of bile from the gall bladder
Cooling	One causing a reduction of temperature and giving rise to feeling of coolness
Demulcent	A compound which soothes and protects the ailimentary canal
Deobstruent	A compound which enables clearing of obstructions in the body and opening the natural passages
Detergent	A substance with cleansing action, internally and externally
Diaphoretic	A substance which stimulates perspiration

Diuretic	A substance increasing the production of urine by stimulating the kidneys
Emetic	A drug which causes one to vomit
Emmenagogue	One that increases menstrual flow
Emmolient	A compound causing the softening and smoothening of skin
Expectorant	A group of drugs which help clearing the respiratory passages by stimulating removal of mucus and other secretions
Febrifuge	One that cause fever to go down
Galactogogue	Compounds stimulating the production and increasing the secretion of breast milk
Hemostatic	One that helps control bleeding
Hepatic	A substance with primary action on the liver
Hydrogogue	A substance with the property of removing water or serum accumulations
Hypnotic	A drug which relaxes and induces sleep
Insecticide	A substance which kills insects
Irritant	A term describing a substance which irritates tissue
Laxative	One that softens stool in order to ease defecation
Mydriatic	A drug which causes the dilation of the pupil
Nervine	Drugs which restore nerves to their original state and function
Narcotic	A substance causing stupor and

	eventual loss of complete consciousness
Nephritic	A drug which has actions on the kidneys
Nutritive	Compounds which nourish the body
Parasiticide	A substance causing elimination of parasites from internal and external body surfaces.
Pectoral	Drugs used in treatment of lung and chest complaints
Purgative	A substance or a measure taken to help evacuate the bowel; this is much more effective than a laxative or an aperient
Refrigerant	A substance producing a feeling of coolness and eliminating thirst
Resolvent	A compound applied to swellings to help reduce them in size
Rubefacient	A compound causing the reddening of skin and hence enabling it to peel off
Sedative	A drug which lessens tension and anxiety; it also calms the nervous system
Sternutatory	A substance which irritates the olfactory nerve endings and stimulates sneezing
Stimulant	Any compound increasing activity of an organ or organ system
Stomachic	A term used to describe drugs which are used to treat stomach disorders
Styptic	Substances which stop bleeding by either contraction of blood vessels

	or rapid clotting of blood
Sudorific	A drug or compound causing profuse perspiration
Taeniacide	Drugs used for expulsion of tapeworms from the body
Tonic	Substances which produce a feeling of wellbeing by imparting strength and vigour to the body
Vermifuge	A compound which kills and expels worms from the intestines
Vesicant	Substance causing blistering when applied to skin
Vulnerary	A drug which has the capacity to heal wounds rapidly

HEALING HERBS

Agrimony-*Agrimonia eupatoria*

Occurrence: Scotland, England

Uses: mild astringent, deobstruent, tonic and diuretic. Excellent for liver problems, skin eruptions, blood diseases as well as snake and insect bites.

Aloes- *Aloe vera*

Occurrence: East and South Africa, West Indies

Uses: antihelminthic, purgative, emmenagogue and vermifuge. Also good for applying on irritated skin

Allspice-*Pimentio officinalis*

Occurrence: West Indies, Jamaica, Central and South America.

Uses: Stimulant, aromatic and carminative, used in case of hysteria and flatulent indigestion.

Anemone, Wood *Anemone nemorosa*

Occurrence: Britain

Uses: headaches, leprosy, lethargy and eye inflammation.

Anemone, Pulsatilla – *Anemone pulsatilla*

Occurrence: limestone areas of Britain

Uses: diaphoretic, antispasmodic and nervine; beneficial for disorders od nervous, respiratory and digestive disorders; specifically used in treatment of bronchitis, asthma and whooping cough.

Angelica- *Angelica archangelica*

Occurrence: Scotland, Lapland and England

Uses: stomachic, diuretic, carminative, stimulant, aromatic, tonic and expectorant; good for colds, rheumatism, pleurisy and wind colic; also good for digestion.

Angostura-*Galipea officinalis*

Occurrence: South America

Uses: purgative, tonic, aromatic, stimulant and bitter; used in bilious diarrhea and dysentery; purgative in action when taken in large doses.

Anise- *Pimpinella anisum*

Occurrence: Egypt, Greece, Crete; Western Asia; central Europe, North Africa

Uses: pectoral and carminative; effective against chest infections and coughs; used to make lozenges; aids digestion; relief catarrh in infants when taken as tea; cathartic and aperient activity, therefore relieves flatulence. It can be used safely during convulsions.

Arrowroot – *Maranta arundinacea*

Occurrence: Central America, Bangladesh, Java, Philippines, Mauritius, West Africa and West Indies

Uses: Non-irritating, demulcent and nutritive; works best with infants with bowel complaints; antibiotic properties; can be used topically on arrow wounds, spider and scorpion bites and to stop gangrene.

Balm-*Melissa officinalis*

Occurrence: Britain

Uses: Febrifuge, carminative, diaphoretic; has a cooling effect when used in tea for patient with fever; used in treatment of cold and fever.

Barley- *Hordeum distichon* and *Hordeum vulgare*

Occurrence: Britain

Uses: nutritive, demulcent; used in feverish patients; barley water is very effective for diarrhea and bowel inflammation in infants.

Basil-*Ocimum basilicum*

Occurrence: Britain

Uses: coolant, aromatic and carminative; used in treatment of nervous disorders; basil infusions are used for intestinal obstruction, nausea and vomiting

Belladonna- *Atropa Belladonna*

Occurrence: Central and southern Europe, England

Uses: anti-spasmodic, narcotic, diuretic, mydriatic; used in coughs, night-fevers and as an anodyne in fever; relieves eye diseases, pain, sciatica, gout and rheumatism; should be used with caution in small amounts as it is poisonous

Bergamot-*Monarda didyma*

Occurrence: North America

Uses: active component is thymol, oil of bergamot used as antispasmodic, carminative, tonic, antiseptic and aromatic; infusion is a good remedy for colds, fever, coughs and sore throat.

Blue-bell-*Scilla nutans*

Occurrence: Western Europe, Britain and Italy.

Uses: styptic, diuretic; excellent medicine for leucorrhea, cure for snake bit. Use dried as fresh bulbs are poisonous.

Borage- *Borago officinalis*

Occurrence: Britain and Europe

Uses: refrigerant, diuretic, emollient, demulcent; acts on kidneys and relieves fevers and pulmonary conditions; used as poultice for inflammatory skin complaints like eczema and psoriasis; flowers eaten raw are source of strength for patients with chronic disease

Broom-*Cytisus scoparius*

Occurrence: Britain, Europe and northern Asia

Uses: Carthtic and diuretic; is an excellent remedy for liver, kidney and bladder disorders once it is given as in infusion with combination of agrimony and dandelion. Must be used carefully as it has strong effects on the heart and can lead to eventual heart failure.

Burdock- *Artium lappa*

Occurrence: England and Europe

Uses: diaphoretic, diuretic and alterative; purifies blood and heals skin conditions; used to treat scurvy, rheumatism and boils, applied in poultice form for bruises, gouty swellings and tumors. Burdock extract is a demulcent and relaxant tonic for skin.

Betterbur-*Petasites vulgaris*

Occurrence: marshy areas in Great Britain

Uses: diuretic, tonic and a cardiac stimulant; remedy for fevers, asthma, plague, urinary complaints and gravel; used in homeopathy for back pain, neuralgia, migraine and painful menstruation. It has proven to be excellent in the treatment of asthma. Recent clinical trials have shown that *petasites* is an effective anti-cancer drug which stopd cancer growth by attacking tumor cells.

Cacao-*Theobroma cacao*

Occurrence: tropical America, Sri Lanka and Java

Uses: nutritive, stimulant, diuretic and emollient. Cocoa butter is used in cosmetics, coating pills and suppositories; excellent moisturizer for hands and feet; *theobromine* has a stimulating effect on the nervous system, much like caffeine and theophylline. It acts on the heart, muscles and kidneys. Useful in heart failure and given in combination with digitalis. Helps lower blood pressure as well.

Camphor-*Cinnamonum camphora*

Occurrence: China, Japan and East Asia

Uses: aromatic, diaphoretic, sedative, anthelminthic, anodyne, antispasmodic. Usually used in chills, colds, fevers, inflammation or diarrhea, taken in cases of nervousness, hysteria and neuralgia. Large doses must be avoided as it has potent effect on the central nervous system.

Caraway-*Carum Carvi*

Occurrence: Britain, Europe and Asia

Uses: carminative, stimulant and aromatic. Used in the treatment of digestive disorders such as dyspepsia, flatulence, and stomach distubances. Excellent when used for infant colic. It is applied in poultice form on bruises. Mostly used as a gourmet flavoring agent.

Cardamom-*Elettaria cardamomum*

Occurrence: Southern India, Sri Lanka

Uses: Aromatic, stimulant and carminative; helpful in indigestion and flatulence, good for colic and headaches. Commonly used as a spice and flavoring agent in Indian food.

Castor oil plant-*Ricinus communis*

Occurrence: India and other tropical and subtropical countries

Uses: Cathartic, purgative, vermifuge, laxative and galactogogue; the last two properties are strongest in this herb, usually effective in children and preganant women; externally applied on ringworm infection, itch and leprosy. Used as a carried oil for drugs such as atropine and cocaine. Industrial uses include soap and varnish manufacturing.

Catmint- *Nepeta cataria*

Occurrence: Zanzibar, Sierra Leone, Japan and Madagascar

Uses: rubefacient, tonic, carminative and stimulant. This is considered as the best and most effective stimulant in herbal medicine. It has naturally warming tendencies which help in blood circulation.

Celery-*Apium graveolens*

Occurrence: Southern Europe, Britain

Uses: Aphrodisiac, nervine, stimulant and carminative; used as a tonic in combination with other herbs, helps promote relaxation, rest, sleep and lack of hysteria. It is also an effective remedy for rheumatism.

Chamomile, *Anthemis nobilis*

Occurrence: British Isles

Uses: Anti-spasmodic, tonic, stomachic, anodyne. Chamomile infusions work wonders with hysteria and nervous disorders, soothing and sedative; mild purgative effective in children and helps as a tonic. Use in poultices for inflammation and bruises. It is useful in relieving toothache and earache.

Chickweed- *Stellania media*

Occurrence: Temperate regions and North Arctic

Uses: refrigerant, demulcent. Used mostly as poultice for healing ulcers and lessening inflammation; more effective in eye and skin conditions.

Chicory-*Cichonium intybus*

Occurrence: England and Ireland

Uses: laxative, diuretic and tonic, beneficial in liver diseases, gout and rheumatism.

Chives-*Allium schoenoprasum*

Occurrence: Northern Europe and Great Britain

Uses: appetite stimulant; aids digestion, treats infections and anemia.

Cinnamon- *Cinnamonum zeylanicum*

Occurrence: Sri Lanka and other eastern countries

Uses: antiseptic, carminative, astringent, aromatic and stimulant. Prevents nausea and vomiting, relieves flatulence and diarrhea; sometimes used to prevent heamorrage of the womb.

Clover, Red-*Trifolium pretense*

Occurrence: Britain and Europe

Uses: antispasmodic, sedative, alterative; excellent for bronchial and whooping cough; very effective as poultice for cancerous growths.

Cloves – *Eugenia carophyllata*

Occurrence: Molucca Islands in southern Phillipines

Uses: aromatic, carminative, stimulant; has volatile oils with strong germicide and antiseptic properties. It is also effective as an expectorant.

Coffee- *Coffea Arabica*

Occurrence: Abyssina and other tropical countries

Uses: anti-emetic, anti-narcotic, stimulant and diuretic; usually used as a beverage. It is a brain stimulant and delays sleep onset; excellent for use in snake bites when preventing patients from falling into a coma; valuable for cardiac disease, fluid retention and diuresis. Also used in the treatment of gout.

Coriander-*Coriandrum sativum*

Occurrence: Southern Europe and Britain

Uses: carminative, aromatic and stimulant. It is a very effective purgative.

Cowslip-*Primula veris*

Occurrence: Wildflowers in Great Britain

Uses: antispasmodic, sedative; relives insomnia and restlessness.

Cumin-*Cuminum cyminum*

Occurrence: Egypt, India, China and Mediterranean countries

Uses: antispasmodic, carminative, stimulant; effective for flatulence, colic and a headache. It can be applied as a plaster on stitches and pains.

Daffodil-*Narcissus pseudo-narcissus*

Occurrence: British Isles, European countries

Uses: anti-emetic, useful in pulmonary catarrh; use cautiously as large doses are toxic to the nervous system; strong astringent properties.

Dandelion-*Taraxacum officinale*

Occurrence: Northern temperate countries

Uses: mild aperient, diuretic, tonic; acts on kidneys and liver, mild laxative; increases appetite and improves digestion. Sometimes it is used in rheumatism and gout.

Dock, Yellow-*Rumex crispus*

Occurrence: Great Britain

Uses: laxative, alterative and tonic; widely used in rheumatism, heamorrhoids and bilious complaints; helpful in blood diseases, scurvy and liver diseases. It is also known to slow down cancer growth; used in treatment of diphtheria.

Eucalyptus-*Eucalyptus globus*

Occurrence: Australia, Tasmania, North and South Africa, India and Southern Europe.

Uses: aromatic, anti-spasmodic, antiseptic, stimulant. It has stimulating effects on the heart; used for its antimalarial properties; also taken in tuberculosis, scarlet fever, intermittent fevers and typhoid.

Evening primrose- *Oenothera biennis*

Occurrence: North America, Britain and Europe

Uses: sedative, astringent; effective in dyspepsia, liver diseases, female pelvic disorders, asthma and whooping cough.

Fennel- *Foeniculum vulgare*

Occurrence: France, Russia, India, Persia and Mediterranean countries.

Uses: stomachic, carminative, aromatic and stimulant; purgative in action; especially effective in digestive disorders.

Fenugreek- *Trigonella foenum graecum*

Occurrence: India, Africa, England and eastern Mediterranean countries

Uses: anti-diabetic; used as poultice for skin infections, abscesses, boils and carbuncles; effective against rickets and anemia.

Foxglove-*Digitalis purpurea*

Occurrence: Great Britain and Europe

Uses: diuretic, sedative and cardiac tonic; stimulates hearts, blood vessels and muscles, raises blood pressure; acts on the kidneys; used in treating epilepsy, internal heamorrhage, delirium tremens and inflammatory conditions. It can be poisonous in high doses. It is an excellent antidote for aconite poisoning, and is administered as a hypodermic injection.

Garlic-*Allium sativum*

Occurrence: Europe, China, South Asia

Uses: stimulant, expectorant, diaphoretic, antiseptic. It is applied as ointment externally for its antiseptic properties. Appropriate for asthma, cough and difficult breathing.

Ginger-*Zingiber officinale*

Occurrence: Asia, West Indies, Jamaica and Africa

Uses: expectorant, carminative and stimulant, very useful in digestive disorders such as dyspepsia, flatulence, gastritis and diarrhea.

Ginseng-*Panax quinquefolium*

Occurrence: China, East Asia, North America, Korea and Japan

Uses: stimulant, tonic, stomachic; excellent for vomiting, nausea, nervous disorders, consumption and exhaustion; stimulates appetite.

Horseradish-*Cochlearia armoracia*

Occurrence: British Isles

Uses: rubefacient, aperient, stimulant, antiseptic, diuretic and diaphoretic. Cleans lung and urinary infections; promotes diuresis; alleviates gout and rheumatism; soothes facial neuralgia, chilblains and rheumatic joints when applied topically. It relives whooping cough and sore throat when taken with vinegar and glycerine. It helps expel worms in children.

Ipecacuanha-*Cephalic ipecacuanha*

Occurrence: Brazil, Bolivia, South America and Europe

Uses: stimulant, diaphoretic, emetic and expectorant; stimulates the stomach, liver, intestines and increases appetite. It is used in amoebic dysentery.

Juniper – *Juniperus communis*

Occurrence: Great Britain

Uses: stomachic, diuretic, carminative; used in kidney and bladder diseases; main use is in dropsy.

Lavender-*Lavandula vera*

Occurrence: mountains of western Mediterranean region, France, Italy and Norway

Uses: nervine, stimulant, carminative and aromatic; tonic against faintness, giddiness, palpitations and colic; relieves neuralgia, sprains and rheumatism. It is widely used in aromatherapy.

Lemon- *Citrus Limonica*

Occurrence: Northern India, Mediterranean countries

Uses: cooling, refrigerant, antiscorbutic, tonic; instant remedy for scurvy, fevers and thirst. It has anti-narcotic properties as well. Makes for a good gargling solution because of astringent properties; cure for severe hiccups; soothing lotion for sunburn; good antimalarial drug and reduces typhoid fever.

Lily of the valley – *Convallaria magalis*

Occurrence: England, Scotland, Europe, North America and Northern Asia

Uses: diuretic, cardiac tonic; similar to foxglove but less potent; recommended in valvular heart disease, dropsy and cardiac failure.

Liquorice-*Glycyrrhiza glabra*

Occurrence: South east Europe, South-west Asia, British Isles

Uses: emollient, demulcent, pectoral, expectorant; remedy for cough and chest complaints; used in lozenges for sore throat and laryngitis.

Marjoram – *Origanum vulgare*

Occurrence: Asia, Europe, North Africa and England

Uses: stimulant, diaphoretic, emmenagogue qualities. It is taken as in infusion and helps bring out spots of measles, produces excessive perspiration; provides relief from spasms, colic and dyspepsia, provides good pain relief for tooth ache.

Marshmallow-*Althaea officinalis*

Occurrence: Europe, England and Scotland

Uses: emollient, demulcent; anti-inflammatory; relieves irritation of alimentary canal and urinary and respiratory organs; effective against bruises, sprains and muscle aches. It is good for chest complaints such as cough and bronchitis.

Myrrh-*Commiphora molmol*

Occurrence: North-East Africa, Arabia

Uses: healing, antiseptic, emmenagogue, astringent, stimulant; used in catarrh, leucorrhea, thrush, athlete's foot, menstrual irregularities. It makes a good gargle for sore throat, ulcers and bleeding gums.

Nettle-*Urtica dioica, Urtica urens*

Occurrence: temperate Europe, Asia, Japan, South Africa and Australia

Uses: anti-asthmatic, diaphoretic, astringent; make a good hair tonic; effective against insomnia.

Olive – *Olea Europea*

Occurrence: Mediterranean countries, Syria, Turkey, Chile, Peru and Australia.

Uses: aperient, laxative, demulcent; used externally for bruises, sprains, rheumatism and cutaneous problems, also effective when used in kidney and chest complaints, plague, chills and fevers.

Pepper – *Piper nigrum*

Occurrence: South India, China, East and West Indies, Malaysia, Philippines, Java, Sumatra and Borneo

Uses: carminative, aromatic, febrifuge and aromatic; remedy for constipation, gonorrhea, prolapsed rectum and works on the urinary system. It has been recommended in paralytic, arthritic, cholera, vertigo and scarlatina disorders.

Peppermint-*Mentha peperita*

Occurrence: Europe, Britain, Asia and America

Uses: antispasmodic, carminative, stimulant, stomachic; used for digestive disorders and cramps. It raises body temperature and induces perspiration.

Rosemary- *Pyrus acuparia*

Occurrence: High altitudes, Britain and Europe

Uses: astringent, diaphoretic, stimulant, tonic, nervine, carminative and stomachic; works well as a hair lotion for baldness and dandruff; used in aromatherapy because of strong fragrance.

Sage-*Salvia officinalis*

Occurrence: northern Mediterranean regions, Britain, France and Germany

Uses: tonic, carminative, stimulant, aromatic and astringent; excellent for gargling with sore throat and bleeding gums; useful against delirium or fevers, nervous diseases, and digestive diseases. Fresh leaves can be rubbed onto teeth for whitening and strengthening gums.

St. John's wort – *Hypericum perforatum*

Occurrence: Britain, Europe, Asia

Uses: resolvent, diuretic, nervine, expectorant and aromatic. It is used in bladder trouble, dysentery, diarrhea and jaundice; good antihelminthic; effective against urinary incontinence; softens hard tissues like tumors; used to sooth heard breasts while breast feeding.

Thyme –*Thymus vulgaris*

Occurrence: Temperate countries in northern Europe

Uses: carminative, tonic, antiseptic, antispasmodic; safe cure from whooping cough, catarrh, wind spasms, colic and fevers. Usually, thyme is used in conjunction with other herbal medicines.

Printed in Great Britain
by Amazon.co.uk, Ltd.,
Marston Gate.